LANEY'S LIST
Recipes That Helped Me Lose Weight!

Written By Elaine Kleid

Published On Amazon

INTRODUCTION

There have been so many inquiries from friends requesting information regarding my personal weight loss journey that I decided to publish a list of recipes that I put together during my weight loss transition. I will highlight a few items that I enjoy using when preparing meals.

I do most of my cooking in coconut oil because it is healthy and has a high heat tolerance. Other oils I enjoy using on occasion are safflower or olive oil or even sesame if I'm in the mood for it.

I prefer to use sea salt in my recipes and I prefer honey in place of sugar in most instances.

Keeping a bag or two of frozen veggies (Kale, Spinach, and a mix of Onions, Peppers & Celery, Broccoli and Brussel Sprouts) is a very convenient way to get fresh veggies anytime!

I don't really drink soda or milk, beer yes, and coffee which I usually drink daily, a very dark roast and black (no cream and no sugar).

Smoothies and peanuts are a great way to get protein fast. If you need to be out the door and don't have a lot of time to cook, grab some peanuts or toss some veggies and fruit in the blender for a quick vitamin boost!

Losing weight for me was not really my focus when I began my weight loss journey. I was profoundly impacted by some information I received so I made the decision to begin eating healthier.

On May 5, 2014 I chose to stop eating meat and chemically ridden foods and as a result I lost about fifty pounds in six months. No gimmicks, no products are endorsing me. This is my personal experience. What prompted me were videos of animal abuse in some of the food production slaughter houses. The videos really affected me. I decided I didn't need to eat meat if that is what I was paying for. I do not judge others that eat meat. I am against the abusive treatment of animals.

That decision, to stop eating meat, caused me to start questioning and reading ingredient labels on foods that I would buy. I decided to stop buying foods with chemicals. For example, if you buy a salad it should read apples, lettuce and carrots if that's what is in there, but if you look on the ingredients label, tell me what you see in that salad mix. So, as a result I buy my lettuce, apples and carrots fresh and separate and then I mix them together myself which takes very little effort or time.

I have been using beans and peanuts for protein and they are quite good. There is a large variety of beans to choose from and there are many different ways to prepare and enjoy them. I keep thinking of new recipes frequently and cannot wait to try them!

I hope you enjoy these recipes as much as I do and I wish you much success on your endeavor to eat healthier!

BREAKFAST RECIPES

Peanut Butter Oatmeal With Banana
(Substitute With Different Nut If Desired)

1 cup of oatmeal
2 Tablespoons of Honey
1 Teaspoon of Cinnamon
1 Banana
Hot water (make to your own preferred consistency)

Egg Omelets With Veggies

1 Tablespoon of Coconut Oil (warm in pan)
2 Eggs
½ Cup of mixed Veggies (onions, peppers and celery)
½ Cup of Kale and or Spinach
Tablespoon minced garlic
½ Roma Tomato
Mozzarella Cheese (your preferred amount)
Salt and Pepper to taste

Enjoy! You can also use a wheat wrap and make a breakfast burrito. And if you brown the wrap first, you'll have a delicious breakfast pizza or even a breakfast enchilada. Don't forget the sour cream. Yum!

Don't be afraid to experiment with your spices. You will discover something new every time! I have even added chili to my egg omelets. Organic chili recipe will be listed later. Beans and eggs are great together. Power packed with protein!

Greek Yogurt (GMO Free)

Greek Yogurt and Pineapple (Fresh Not Canned) Delicious! Add walnuts, almonds, pistachios or peanuts or a nut of your choice for protein power!

SMOOTHIES

These Combos Taste Great! Nuts are also a great addition of protein and flavor. Experiment!

Spinach, Strawberry, Greek Yogurt, Orange, Cucumber

Spinach, Pineapple, Greek Yogurt, Tomato, Cucumber

Spinach, Apple, Pineapple, Banana, Greek Yogurt

Spinach, Banana, Apple, Greek Yogurt, Strawberry

SNACK RECIPES

Cheese and Crackers With Fruit

Vegetable crackers
Cheese (Mozzarella, White Cheddar)
1 sliced apple
The salty, sweet alternating of flavors make this snack very interesting. I like to alternate between bites of cheese and cracker and then apple.

ON THE GO SNACKS

Peanuts

(Read the label for ingredients to read Peanuts and Salt) That's all that should be in the container. I make an attempt to avoid any that have other oils in them. I like to keep some with me in a zip lock bag so when I am out and I get hungry then I have them on hand.

Almonds

Almonds are also a very healthy snack and portable in a zip lock bag so if you don't like peanuts these are a great alternative.

Pumpkin Seeds

These I eat with the shell on. The ingredients should also read pumpkin seeds and salt and that should be all that is listed in the ingredients.

Baby Carrots

Baby carrots are a great snack if you are in a hurry and don't have time to prep anything. You can just grab a handful and walk out the door. I usually pass a few out to the dogs and goats along the way because they enjoy them too!

LUNCH RECIPES

Traditional Garden Salad

I prefer organic spinach leaves or Romaine lettuce.
½ Roma Tomato
Cheese (white cheeses like cream cheese, mozzarella or white cheddar (Use chunked white cheddar, not shredded)
Green olives
Cucumbers
Sea Salt and Black Pepper to your preference.

Homemade Potato Salad

When I make potato salad at home I use potatoes boiled with the skin on and add mustard that has turmeric in it because I have read of some health benefits. Then I season and flavor according to what I am craving. Here are the main ingredients I use.

3 Large Potatoes
2 Tablespoons of Koops Spicy Mustard (or organic mustard)
1 Cup Mixed Veggies (celery, onions, peppers)
1 Tablespoon Black Pepper
1 Tablespoon Sea Salt
1/3 Tub or Stonyfield Greek Yogurt (No GMO or High Fructose Corn Syrup)
1 Small Tub of Sour Cream

Make it as creamy as you like. I sometimes like to add green olives and roasted red peppers. I am considering adding a couple boiled eggs to try in the near future. Sounds yummy!

Cucumber Salad

1 Cucumber
3 slices of Onion
½ Roma Tomato
2 Tablespoon Sour Cream
1 Tteaspoon Organic Catsup
1 Teaspoon of Spicy Brown Mustard (I like the Koops brand because it contains Tumeric, Vinegar, Water, Mustard Seed and Salt)
Black Pepper

Egg Salad

Hard Boiled Eggs
Sour cream and Cream Cheese mixed (Instead of mayo)
Salt and Pepper
Add celery or other veggies if you want
Explore! Tasty!

Bean and Cheese Burrito

You can add sour cream and cream cheese to make a
creamy flavorful sauce.

Refried Beans (Pile them on!)
Mozzarella Cheese (as much as you want)
Sour Cream
Cream Cheese
Tomato (Fresh veggies are always good!)
Mixed Veggies (Onions, Peppers and Celery)
Pepper and Salt to your preference
Wheat Wrap

DINNER RECIPES

Wheat Wrap Pizzas

These are a great dinner and are ready within about 15 minutes. You can flavor them to your liking just like a personal pizza. If you feel like Mexican, add some Cumin, if you feel like Indian, add some Curry or if you want spicy add some hot sauce! Bring on the spice!

Wheat Wrap
Mozzarella Cheese
Refried Beans (Traditional which has no preservatives)
Mixed Veggies (onions, celery, peppers, frozen precut)
Spinach Leaves Fresh or Frozen
Fresh Tomato
Garlic Minced
Sour Cream (after toasting in a toaster oven or conventional oven)
Seasonings of your choice

Organic Chili

1 Small Bag of Raw Red Beans (Pink Beans are also good)
2 cups Spinach or Kale
2 cups Mixed Veggies (Onions, Peppers, Celery)
1 can of Refried Beans (add after boiling beans and veggies)
1 jar or Organic Spaghetti Sauce (Or Organic Marinara)
10 Brussel Sprouts (A healthy alternative to meatballs)
1 Tablespoon Minced Garlic
2 Tablespoons of Chili Powder
Salt and Pepper to your preference

Boil the beans for about an hour.
Add the veggies and cook on medium low for about 10-15 minutes.
Add the refried beans (drain veggies if there is a considerable amount of water. Otherwise it is okay to leave the water in there to retain the full flavor of all of the vegetables).
Add the jar of spaghetti sauce
Add the Chili Powder
Season the chili to your own preference. Sea Salt, Honey and some Black Pepper make a great combo!

For those of you that like to eat spicy, (I am a huge spicy fan) try adding a hot pepper to the veggies when you put them in to boil. I love habanero peppers but Serrano peppers and jalapeno peppers are also a good addition to give this dish a tasty kick! It's also great to experiment because you get new flavors every time. New ideas will just start to flow. "What would it taste like if I added this?" Is one of the questions that I have been asking myself and am experiencing new flavors and loving it. Be Brave!

Chili Leftovers? Here's An Idea

I find that the leftover chili is fantastic with scrambled eggs. Spicy or not it is a great new flavor that I very much enjoy! Experiment and try it with something else you like. You just may be surprised at how good it tastes!

Organic Meatless Spaghetti or Goulash

½ Box Veggie Pasta (Not enriched white)
2 Cups Kale
2 Cups Mixed Veggies (Onions, Peppers, Celery)
1 Can Traditional Refried Beans
1 Jar of Organic Spaghetti Sauce (Or Organic Marinara)
1 Tablespoon Minced Garlic
10 Brussel Sprouts

I like to boil the veggie noodles for a few minutes then add the frozen veggie mix and kale. If you make the water level just about an inch above the noodles then you will not have to strain them at all. The frozen vegetables will be ready in about 5 minutes and then you can add the can of refried beans and the sauce and viola! Have some bread and butter on the side, in moderation of course. The bean are a protein booster and the flavor is very good when mixed with the sauce. I love to add the brussel sprouts to make it look like meatballs and my husband loves it.

Bean Burgers

1 Can Traditional Refried Beans
½ Cup Mixed Veggies (Celery, Onions, Peppers)
1 Tablespoon Minced Garlic
1 Teaspoon Cumin
1 Teaspoon Cajun Spice
1 Teaspoon Curry
1 Tablespoon Turmeric (Or Spicy Mustard that contains it)
1 Teaspoon Sea Salt
1 Teaspoon Black Pepper
2 Cups Oatmeal
1 Jumbo Egg
3 Tablespoons Coconut Oil (Place Oil In A Frying Pan)
2 Pieces Toast

With the exception of the egg and coconut oil, mix all the other ingredients together and taste test to see if you want to add something else. The key is to create a flavor that you like, so experiment, that's part of the fun!

Once flavored to your liking, add the egg and stir well. Place the coconut oil in a large frying pan and set the stove burner on medium high heat and then pour the mixture into the frying pan. Cook until the bottom starts to get crispy then flip over the mixture in sections and cook for another few minutes. (This will not necessarily stick together which is fine because it will still hold well on the toast when you make your sandwich) After the other side is browning well, stir and let it cook until it is as crispy as you would like it to be. Remove from heat, toast your bread and make your sandwich! (I like to add organic ketchup to my sandwich) Add cheese if you want to! Delicious!

Bean Frita

1 Can Traditional Refried Beans
½ Cup Mixed Veggies (Celery, Onions, Peppers)
1 Tablespoon Minced Garlic
1 Tablespoon Turmeric (Or Spicy Mustard that contains it)
1 Teaspoon Sea Salt
1 Teaspoon Black Pepper
2 Cups Oatmeal
2 Jumbo Eggs
6 Tablespoons Coconut Oil
1 Cup Flour

Place the mixed ingredients into a 9 X 11 or 9 X 13 inch baking dish and put it in the oven. Set the temperature to 375 and let bake for about 15 minutes, check to see how it's doing and then finish cooking it until it is as brown as you would like it to be.

Add cheese to the top toward the end of baking time and top with fresh tomato. Mmmm Mmmm Good!

Add a garden salad to the side for a great accompaniment. And don't forget the sour cream!

Organic Creamy Tomato Soup

5 Roma Tomatoes
1 Small Tub of Sour Cream
1 Teaspoon Oregano
½ Cup Sauteed Mixed Veggies (Onions, Celery, Peppers)
½ Teaspoon Sea Salt
½ Teaspoon Black Pepper

Blend everything except the mix veggies. Then add all the ingredients into a saucepan. Heat the ingredients in the saucepan on medium. Stir it kind of frequently to make sure that it doesn't stick to the pan.

Now you can either put on your favorite grilled cheese sandwich to accompany your soup or you can use this same recipe as a delicious pasta sauce! I have even used it to top my personal tortilla pizzas!

Split Pea and Potato Soup

5 Large Potatoes
1 Bag of Dried Split Peas
2 Cups Mixed Veggies (Onions, Peppers, Celery)
Baby Carrots (You decide how many you want in there)
Salt and Pepper to your taste preference

Boil the potatoes (skin on) and the bag of split peas together for about an hour and then add the mixed frozen veggies (onions, green peppers and celery). Add the baby carrots and cook on medium low until the carrots are soft and the soup should thicken. Once it reaches your desired consistency, it's ready!

Curried Black Eyed Pea Soup With Kale

1 Bag of Black Eyed Peas
2 Cups of Kale
2 Cups Mixed Veggies (Onions, Peppers, Celery)
2 Tablespoons of Curry (Add more or less to your liking)
1 Tablespoon Minced Garlic
1 Teaspoon Sea Salt
1 Teaspoon Black Pepper

This is a simple recipe I recently created. You can mix everything together once the black eyed peas are boiled (for about an hour) and soft. I add a little more water to cover about an inch above the entire contents after adding the vegetables and seasonings and then I cook it on medium and check it about every half hour or so until it reaches my desired consistency.

Soup Accompaniment
Bean Bread

4 Cups of flour
1 Can of Traditional Refried Beans
2 Tablespoons Coconut Oil
2 Tablespoons Organic Spicy Mustard or Turmeric
1 Teaspoon Salt
2 Teaspoons Sugar
1 Teaspoon Black Pepper

Mix and bake at 350 for 40 minutes in a 9 X 5 baking dish.

DESSERTS

Chocolate Cake

1 Large Bar 100% Cacao
½ Cup Coconut Oil
2 Eggs
2 Cups Sugar
2 Cups Self Rising Flour
½ Teaspoon Sea Salt
½ Teaspoon Baking Soda
1 Teaspoon Cinnamon
½ Cup Organic Cream, Sour Cream or Greek Yogurt
(If you do not want to use dairy, you can use water)

Mix all of the ingredients together in a bowl. If you find the mixture is dryer than you prefer, you can add 1-2 tablespoons more of coconut oil, water or cream (your preference). Grease a 9 X 13" cake pan with coconut oil and pour the cake mix into the pan.

Cook in the preheated oven at 350 degrees for about 30 minutes and place a toothpick or butter knife in the center to see if anything sticks to it. If there is cake stuck to the toothpick or the butter knife then cook another 10 minutes and repeat until the knife comes out clean.

I do not like to frost my cakes due to the amount of sugar that is already in them.

Pineapple Coconut Tropical Cake

This cake is delicious!

2 Cups Fresh Pineapple (chunked small)
½ Cup Coconut Oil
2 Eggs
2 Cups Sugar
2 Cups Self Rising Flour
½ Teaspoon Sea Salt
½ Teaspoon Baking Soda
1 Teaspoon Cinnamon

Mix all of the ingredients together in a bowl. If you find the mixture is dryer than you prefer, you can add 1-2 tablespoons more of coconut oil. There should be plenty of juice from the pineapple to keep this cake mixture moist. Grease a 9 X 13" cake pan with coconut oil and pour the cake mix into the pan. Sprinkle the top with coconut flakes and maybe a couple teaspoons of sugar.

Place the cake in the preheated oven and cook at 350 degrees for about 30 minutes and place a toothpick or butter knife in the center to see if anything sticks to it. If there is cake stuck to the toothpick or the butter knife then cook another 10 minutes and repeat until the knife comes out clean.

MORNING METABOLISM BOOST
Drink at least one hour before having coffee.

1 Glass of Water
1 Teaspoon Apple Cider Vinegar
1 Teaspoon Honey
1 Teaspoon Lemon Vinegar

I also like to add lemon vinegar that I make by putting a cut up lemon into white vinegar for 2 weeks. You can use it anytime really but I am pretty sure that 2 weeks is the standard fermentation period when placing fruits and veggies in vinegar.

If you prefer more honey, then add another teaspoon or better yet add more water instead and keep the calorie intake low.

THANK YOU!

Thank you to everyone that has been cheering me on! These recipes should keep you busy for a little while. I hope that you will post your pictures or share your story with me on your successful weight loss journey. Modifying the types of food you choose to eat will greatly impact your weight very quickly. I wish you much success! Cheers!

www.ingramcontent.com/pod-product-compliance
Lightning Source LLC
Chambersburg PA
CBHW062034280526
45787CB00005B/2315